GREEN DETOX SMOOTHIES FOR GLAUCOMA

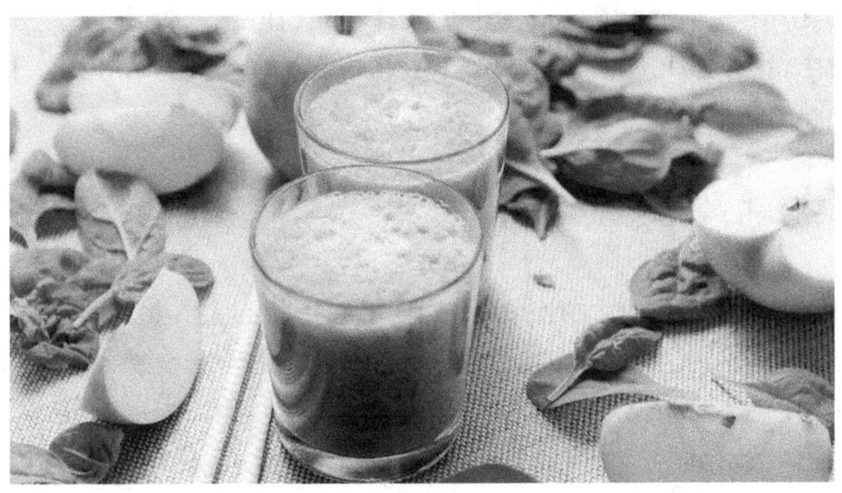

Easy & Effective Natural Detoxifying Recipes for Glaucoma Relief and Overall Wellnes

Dr Ikukoyi Oluwaseun Akintan

Copyright

ISBN: 9798323302796

The information provided in this book is designed to provide helpful insights on the subjects discussed. This book is not meant to be used, nor should it be used, to diagnose or treat any medical condition. For diagnosis or treatment of any medical problem, consult your physician. The publisher and author are not responsible for any specific health or allergy needs that may require medical supervision and are not liable for any damages or negative consequences from any treatment, action, application or preparation, to any person reading or following the information in this book.

Dedication

This book is dedicated to the Creator of the universe, who gives us all things to enjoy freely.

Also, to every glaucoma patient striving to maintain their remaining vision.

Disclaimer

Dear Reader,

Kindly read the following disclaimers and ensure you understand them before proceeding.

1. This book is not intended to be a research paper, so, I have not included any research work.

2. I deliberately want to make it as short and succinct as possible, to keep readers interested and to avoid boredom.

3. Please don't be offended if you find any typo. However, I have tried as much as possible to avoid that.

4. Medical Advice: The information provided in this book is for educational purposes only and should not be considered a substitute for professional medical advice, diagnosis, or treatment. It is essential to consult with a qualified healthcare professional before making any decisions regarding your eye health.

5. Individual Results: The techniques and recommendations mentioned in this book may vary in effectiveness from person to person. While some individuals may experience positive results, others may not. It is important to understand that everyone's eye health is unique, and outcomes may differ.

6. Personal Responsibility: The author and publisher of this book are not responsible for any adverse effects, injuries, or damages that may arise from the implementation of the techniques or recommendations provided. It is your responsibility to use your judgment and consult a healthcare professional before making any changes to your eye care routine.

Table of Contents

Copyright   ii

Dedication   iii

Disclaimer   iv

Table of Contents   v

INTRODUCTION   1
In the Blink of an Eye: A Tale of Glaucoma

CHAPTER ONE   3
THE GROWING TREND OF ALTERNATIVE TREATMENTS FOR GLAUCOMA

CHAPTER TWO   5
Understanding Glaucoma: From an Ophthalmologist's Perspective

CHAPTER THREE   7
The Role of Nutrition in Eye Health

CHAPTER FOUR   9
GREEN DETOX SMOOTHIES RECIPES

Blueberry and Kale Vision Booster Smoothie   10

Spinach and Pineapple Eye Elixir Smoothie   11

Celery and Apple Eye Soother Smoothie   12

Broccoli and Blueberry Eye Supporter Smoothie   13

Cucumber & Kiwi Eye Booster Smoothie   14

Carrot & Beetroot Eye Cleanser Smoothie   15

Tangy Spinach Salad with Mangos   16

Berrylicious Blast Smoothie   17

Tropical Green Dream Smoothie   18

Spinach and Pineapple Eye Revitalizer Smoothie   19

Eye-Bright Booster Smoothie   20

Beetroot Berry Blast Smoothie   21

Green Power Smoothie   22

Citrus Sunshine Smoothie   23

Ginger Zinger Smoothie   24

Tropical Turmeric Twist Smoothie   25

Superfood Seed Surprise Smoothie   26

About the Author   28

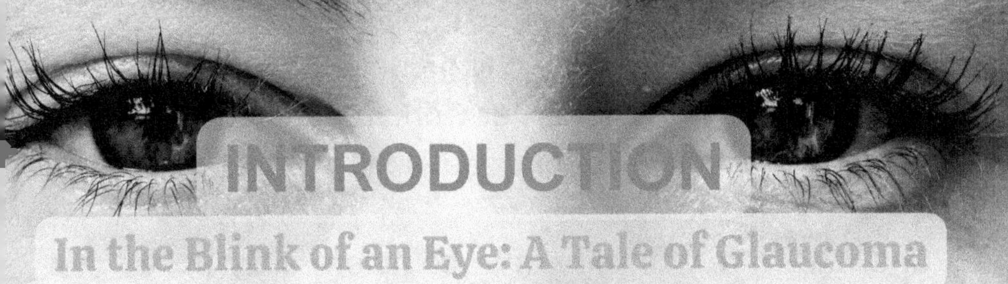

There was once a young woman named Lily. She was a bright, ambitious graduate who aspired to become a well-known architect. Her designs were unique, and her enthusiasm for her work was clear to everyone who knew her.

However, Lily was diagnosed with glaucoma at a young age. Despite the diagnosis, she had a limited understanding of the disease's severity and probable impact on her life. She was frequently too preoccupied with her academics and employment to keep up with her eye appointments and medication schedule.

One day, while working on a blueprint for a prominent architectural competition, Lily noticed her vision going fuzzy. She disregarded it as weariness and kept working long hours, ignoring the warning signs.

Her vision deteriorated quickly over time, and she gradually lost the ability to perceive the exquisite intricacies of her drawings. She eventually sought medical attention, but it was too late. Her glaucoma had developed substantially, and she had lost her vision entirely.

Her blindness has far-reaching consequences. Lily was no longer able to pursue her work in architecture, which demanded a high level of visual acuity.

She had to rely on others to complete daily duties that she had previously taken for granted. Her dreams were destroyed, and she plunged into a deep depression.

The consequences of Lily's blindness went beyond her personal life. Society lost a young architect whose innovative concepts had the potential to reshape cityscapes. The healthcare system suffered additional costs for her recovery and mental health care. Her relatives and friends experienced emotional distress as they witnessed their loved one struggle.

Lily's tale is a sobering reminder of the devastation caused by glaucoma when not properly controlled. It emphasizes the significance of frequent eye examinations, adherence to therapy, and public knowledge of the disease.

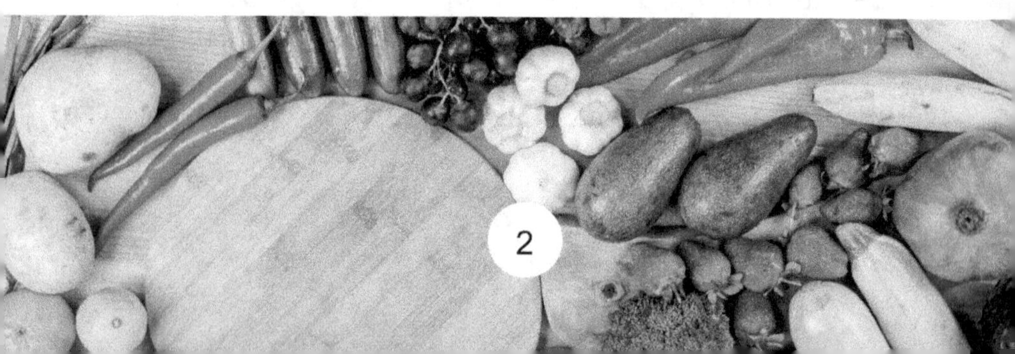

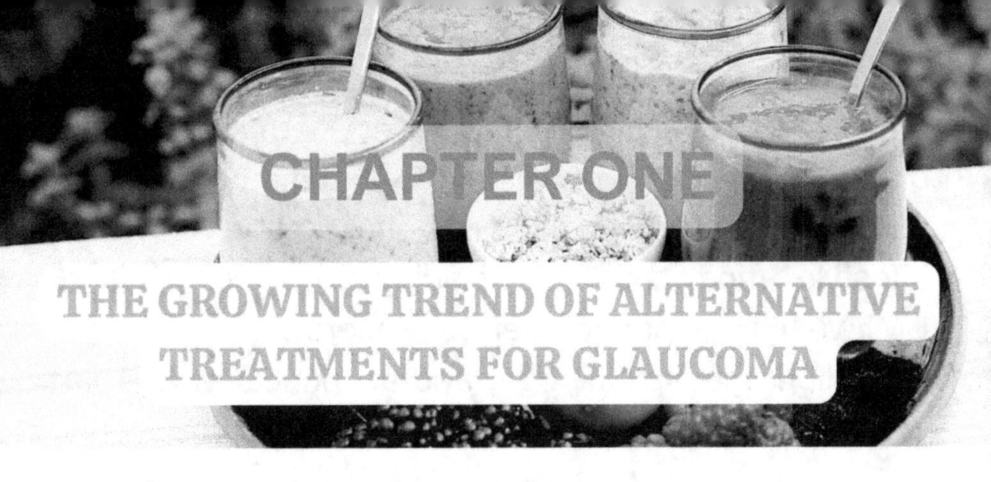

THE GROWING TREND OF ALTERNATIVE TREATMENTS FOR GLAUCOMA

Alternative glaucoma treatments are becoming more widespread, with at least one-third of patients utilizing them. Here are some of the increasing trends:

Vitamins and supplements: Vitamins are one of the most popular and commonly available alternative treatments because of their established benefits and simplicity of access. Vitamins A, C, B9, and B12 offer antioxidant properties. Omega-3 fatty acids are known to have anti-inflammatory and antioxidant benefits on the eye. Dark leafy greens, which contain high quantities of vitamins A, C, and K and nitrate, are also ingested.

Cannabis has been studied in glaucoma because it causes a short-term drop in intraocular pressure (IOP). However, the drug's benefits last only 3 or 4 hours, and a high level of cannabis substances must be maintained inside the patient's system to have a long-term benefit.

Homeopathic treatments have neuroprotective and antioxidant effects on the eye, perhaps slowing glaucoma progression. The most common of these cures are bilberry and ginkgo biloba.

Lifestyle modifications, including sleeping position, BMI/weight management, exercise, smoking cessation, meditation/yoga, and acupuncture, are part of an alternative therapeutic strategy.

New Medications and Surgeries: Patients now have access to new types of glaucoma medications, and the use of selective laser trabeculoplasty (SLT) as a first-line treatment is becoming more common. Several new, safer surgical methods in the "micro-invasive glaucoma surgery" (MIGS) category have altered the traditional landscape of glaucoma treatment.

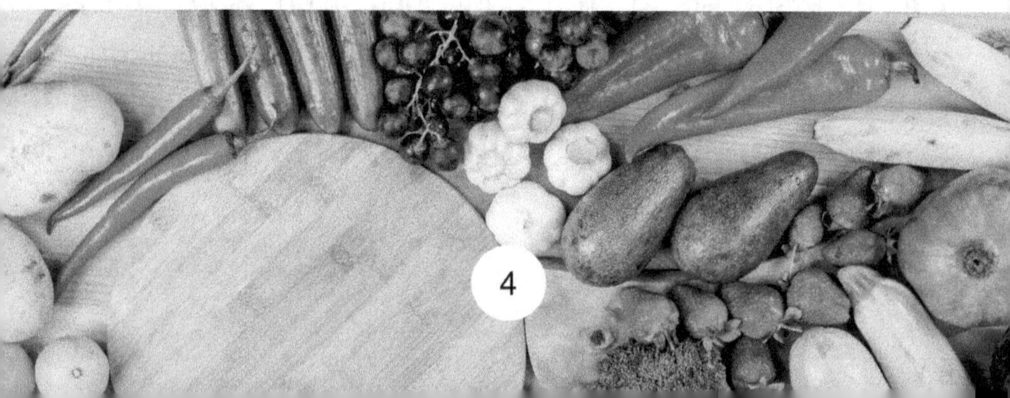

CHAPTER TWO

Understanding Glaucoma: From an Ophthalmologist's Perspective

Glaucoma is a complex condition that affects millions of individuals worldwide and is one of the primary causes of irreversible vision loss. It is defined by optic nerve injury, which is frequently associated with high intraocular pressure (IOP) but can also occur at normal IOP levels.

Types of Glaucoma

Glaucoma is classified into two types: primary open angle glaucoma (POAG) and angle-closure glaucoma (ACG). POAG, the most prevalent type, is a slow-progressing condition that frequently goes unrecognized until considerable vision loss occurs. ACG, on the other hand, might occur unexpectedly and is considered a medical emergency.

Risk Factors:

Glaucoma is caused by a combination of risk factors, including age, family history, race, excessive myopia, hypertension, and diabetes.

Regular eye examinations are essential for early detection, particularly for people who have certain risk factors.

Pathophysiology

The pathophysiology of glaucoma is complex and poorly understood. It is hypothesized to be caused by an imbalance in aqueous humor production and drainage, which results in elevated IOP.

This pressure can injure the optic nerve, causing vision loss. However, some persons may develop optic nerve damage at low pressures, indicating that other variables are at play.

Symptoms and diagnosis

Glaucoma is usually asymptomatic until considerable visual loss occurs. This is why it is known as the "sneak thief of sight". A full eye exam, which includes IOP assessment, optic nerve examination, and visual field testing, is often used to make the diagnosis.

Treatment

The goal of glaucoma treatment is to reduce IOP to a level that will prevent additional optic nerve damage. This is frequently accomplished with eye medications, laser therapy, or surgery. It is crucial to emphasize that these treatments can help prevent additional eyesight loss, but they cannot restore it.

Conclusion

Understanding glaucoma is critical for early diagnosis and treatment. Regular eye exams are essential, particularly for people with risk factors. While there is no cure for

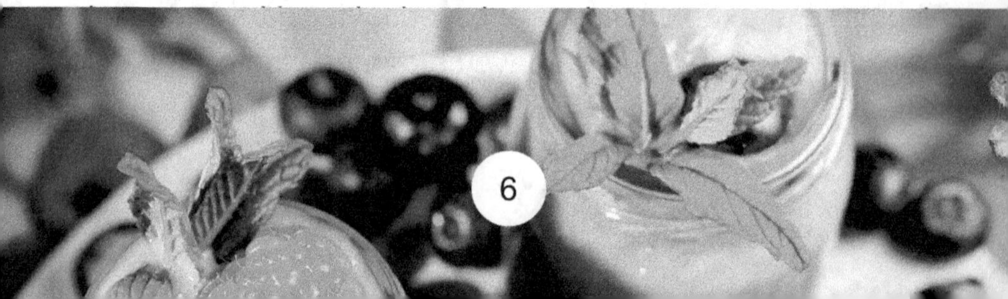

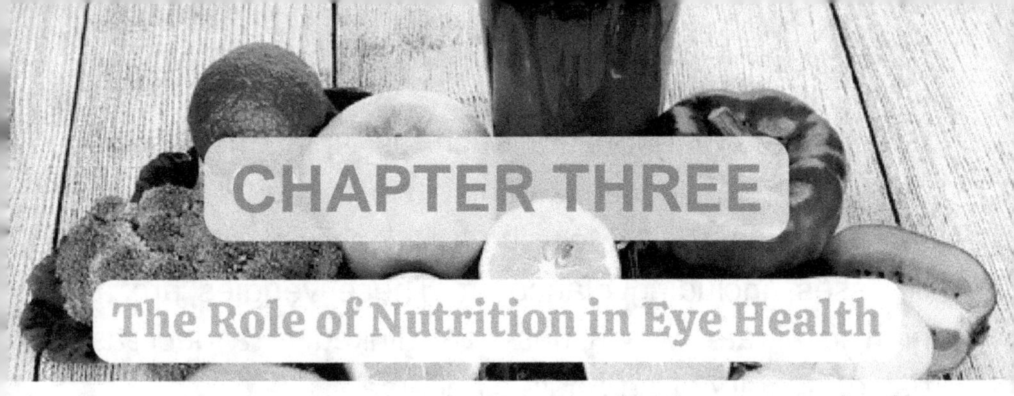

As an Optometrist, I cannot emphasize enough the importance of proper nutrition in sustaining eye health. A well-balanced diet can help avoid several eye problems, including glaucoma.

Nutrition and Ocular Health

The eyes are complicated organs that require a wide range of nutrients to function properly. Antioxidants such as vitamins A, C, and E, as well as minerals like zinc and selenium, are very beneficial to eye health. These nutrients assist to protect the eyes from oxidative stress, which is a destructive process that can affect our cells, including those in our eyes.

Diet and Glaucoma

When it comes to glaucoma, research has shown that certain nutrients can improve eye health and potentially decrease the disease's progression.

For example, antioxidants can help protect the optic nerve from injury. Omega-3 fatty acids, found in fish and flaxseeds, have anti-inflammatory qualities and may help lower intraocular pressure, a risk factor for glaucoma.

Green leafy vegetables

Green leafy vegetables, such as spinach and kale, contain lutein and zeaxanthin, two nutrients that have been shown to reduce the incidence of chronic eye illnesses, including glaucoma. These veggies are also high in nitrate, which has been linked to a decreased risk of primary open-angle glaucoma.

Hydration

Proper hydration is essential for eye health. Drinking enough of water will help you maintain fluid balance in your eyes and avoid dry eye problems.

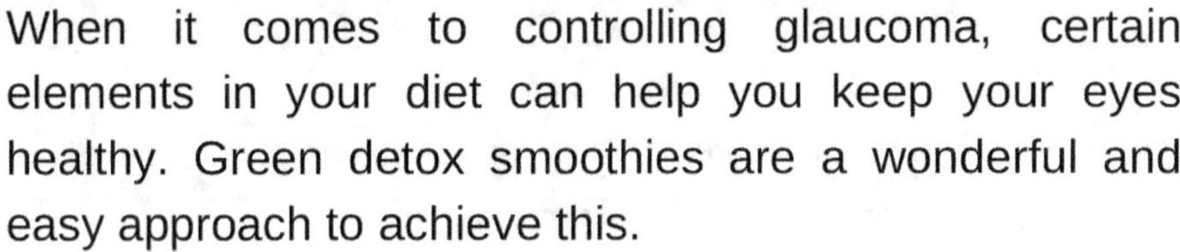

When it comes to controlling glaucoma, certain elements in your diet can help you keep your eyes healthy. Green detox smoothies are a wonderful and easy approach to achieve this.

Why Green Detox Smoothies?

Green detox smoothies contain plenty of leafy greens and fruits, making them a nutrient-dense meal or snack. They include a high concentration of vitamins, minerals, and antioxidants, which can benefit overall health, including vision.

Key Nutrients for Glaucoma.

As I earlier mentioned, certain nutrients are especially beneficial to persons with glaucoma:

Vitamins: A, C, B9, and B12. These vitamins contain potent antioxidants that can help protect the eyes from harm. They can be found in a variety of fruits and vegetables, making them an easy addition to smoothies.

Omega-3s: These fatty acids are anti-inflammatory and may help lower intraocular pressure, which is a risk factor for glaucoma. Flaxseeds and chia seeds are great plant-based sources of Omega-3s and can be readily incorporated into smoothies.

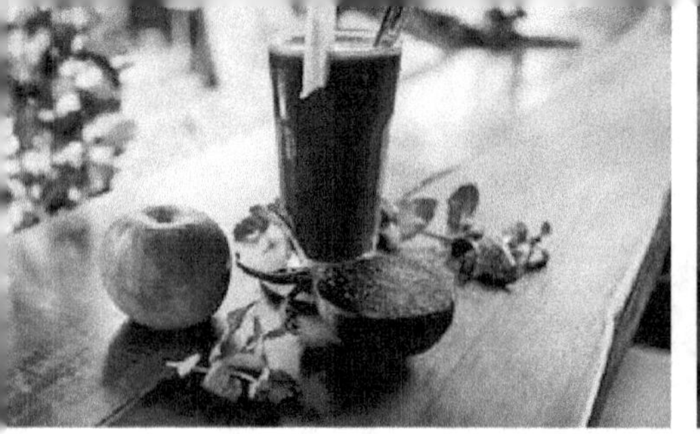
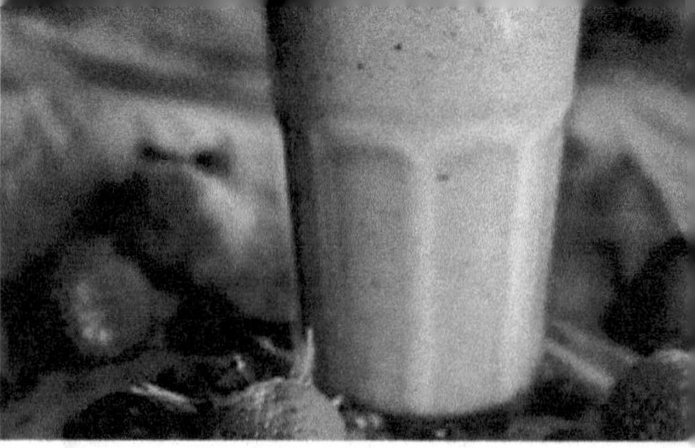

Blueberry and Kale Vision Booster Smoothie

 Vegan 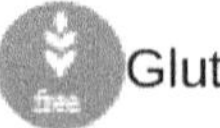 Gluten free 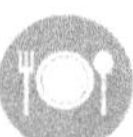 4 Servings 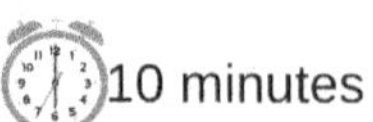 10 minutes

INGREDIENTS

- 2 cups freshly chopped kale leaves
- 1 cup frozen or fresh blueberries for antioxidants.
- 1 ripe banana, peeled and sliced precisely
- 1 tablespoon ground flaxseeds for omega-3 benefits
- For a touch of sweetness, add 1 tablespoon honey.
- 1 1/2 cups of coconut water for hydration and smooth consistency.

DIRECTIONS

1. In a blender, combine kale, blueberries, banana, flaxseeds, honey, and coconut water.

2. Blend the ingredients on high speed until smooth and creamy, making sure all components are fully combined.

3. Pour the smoothie into glasses and serve immediately to enjoy the fresh flavors and nutrients at their best

4. Consume this nutrient-dense combo on a regular basis to promote eye health.

This brilliant green smoothie is a nutrient powerhouse. Every sip delivers antioxidants, vitamins, and minerals!

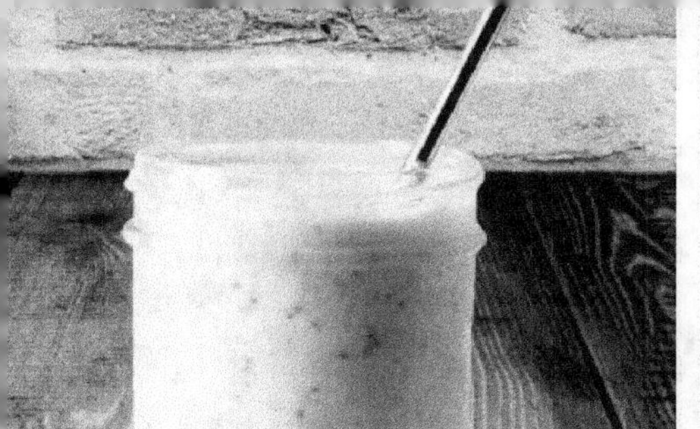 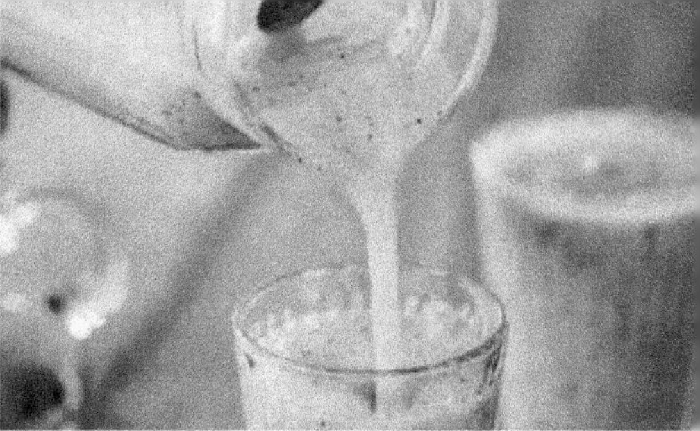

Spinach and Pineapple Eye Elixir Smoothie

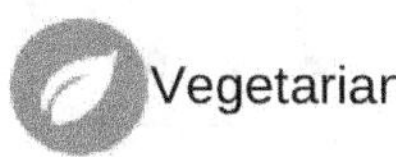 Vegetarian 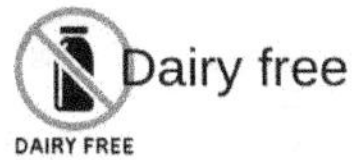 Dairy free 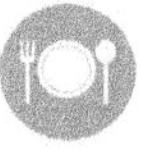 4 Servings 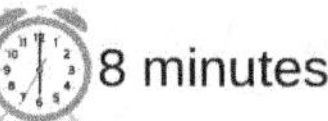 8 minutes

INGREDIENTS

- Wash and dry 2 cups of spinach.
- Add 1 cup of fresh or frozen pineapple pieces for a tropical flavor.
- Peel and slice 1/2 cucumber carefully.
- Add 1 tablespoon of chia seeds for omega-3 fatty acids.
- 1 teaspoon freshly grated fresh ginger
- 1 cup coconut milk for creamy texture

DIRECTIONS

1. Blend spinach, pineapple pieces, cucumber slices, chia seeds, ginger, and coconut milk.

2. Combine the ingredients and blend until smooth and creamy, achieving a consistent texture.

3. Pour the smoothie into glasses and top with a piece of cucumber or pineapple for a bit of freshness.

4. Add this eye-boosting smoothie to your diet on a daily basis to reap the benefits of the nutrients it contains for good eye and general health.

This delightful green elixir contains critical nutrients that nourish your eyes and improve general well-being.

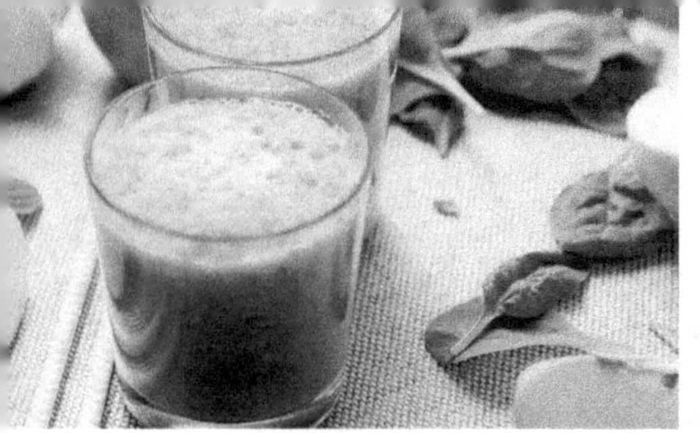
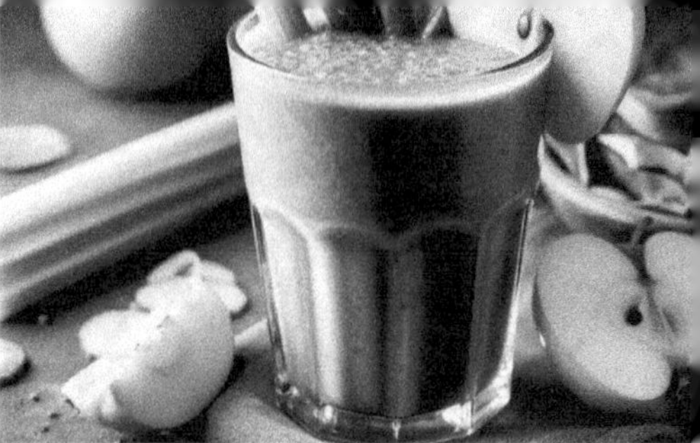

Celery and Apple Eye Soother Smoothie

Vegetarian  *Gluten-free* 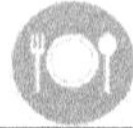4 Servings 7 minutes

INGREDIENTS

- 3 stalks of celery, washed and chopped with care.
- 2 green apples, cored and sliced.
- 1/2 cucumber, peeled and diced.
- 1 tablespoon of fresh mint leaves.
- 1 tablespoon of lemon juice, freshly squeezed.
- 1 cup of water

DIRECTIONS

1. In a blender, combine celery, green apples, cucumber, mint leaves, lemon juice, and water.
2. Blend the mixture until smooth, ensuring that all components are fully combined.
3. Pour the smoothie into cups and serve chilled for a refreshing drink.
4. Drink this eye-soothing smoothie on a daily basis to reap the benefits of its refreshing components, which enhance eye health. Incorporate this blend into your daily routine to benefit your eyes.

This green smoothie soothing. Enjoy the refreshing influence of celery and mint in this delectable recipe.

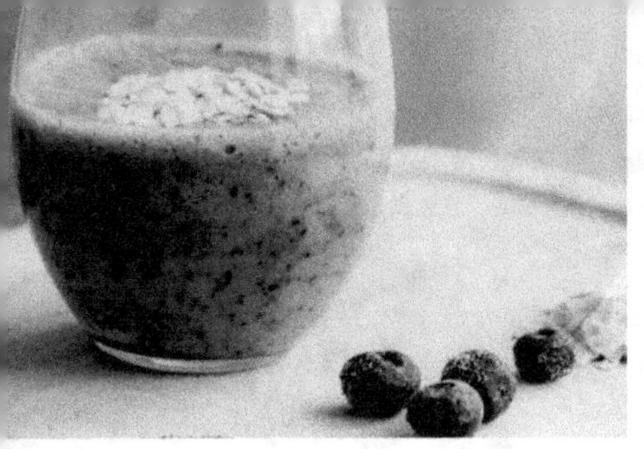
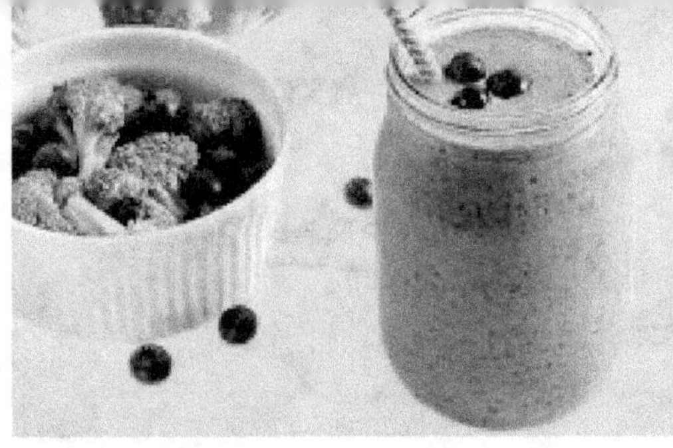

Broccoli and Blueberry Eye Supporter Smoothie

 Vegetarian 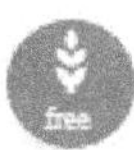 Gluten free 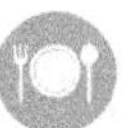 2 Servings 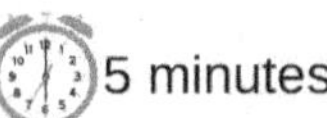 5 minutes

INGREDIENTS

- 1 cup broccoli florets

- 1/2 cup blueberries.

- 1 chopped celery stalk

- 1 tablespoon chia seeds.

- 1 cup of coconut water.

DIRECTIONS

1. Combine all of Broccoli, Blueberries, celery stalk and Chia seeds in a blender

2. Blend the mixture until smooth, ensuring that all components are fully combined.

3. Pour the coconut water and blend for another minute for proper mixing

.

4. Serve in cup and consume immediately.

This smoothie is high in antioxidants and minerals that promote eye health.

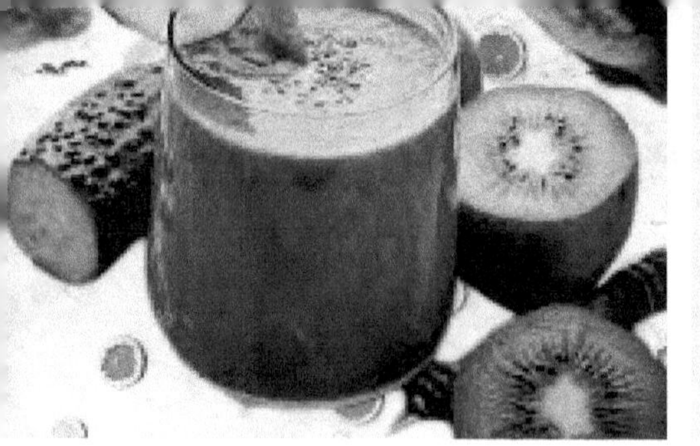
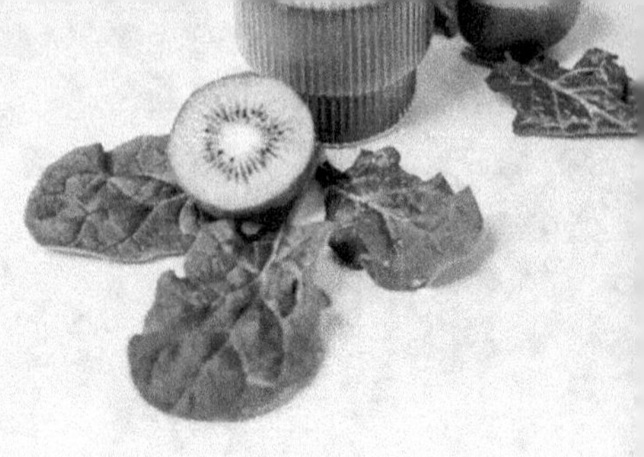

Cucumber & Kiwi Eye Booster Smoothie

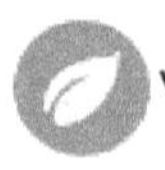 Vegan 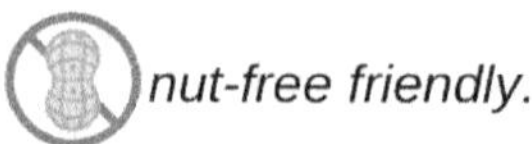 *nut-free friendly.*  2 Servings  5 minutes

INGREDIENTS

- 1/2 cucumber, peeled and sliced

- 2 kiwis, peeled and diced

- 1/2 avocado, peeled and pitted

- 1 tablespoon honey

- 1 cup coconut water

Each sip promises hydration and a bounty of key minerals essential for maintaining eye health.

DIRECTIONS

1. Begin with the cool, crisp essence of 1/2 a cucumber, peeled and sliced,

2. Introduce the vibrant zing of 2 kiwis, peeled and diced,

3. Add 1/2 an avocado, peeled and pitted, its buttery flesh blending seamlessly into the mix.

4. Drizzle in a tablespoon of honey, nature's liquid gold, adding a touch of natural sweetness that complements the fresh flavors.

5. Finally, pour in a cup of coconut water, infusing the concoction with its subtle tropical notes and electrolytes,

6. Blend these ingredients to a velvety smoothness

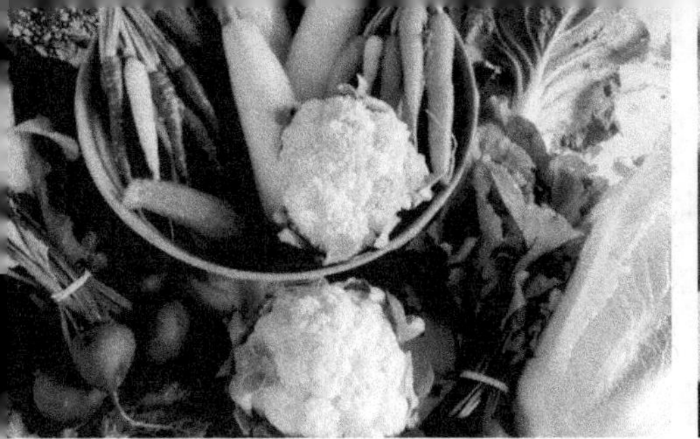
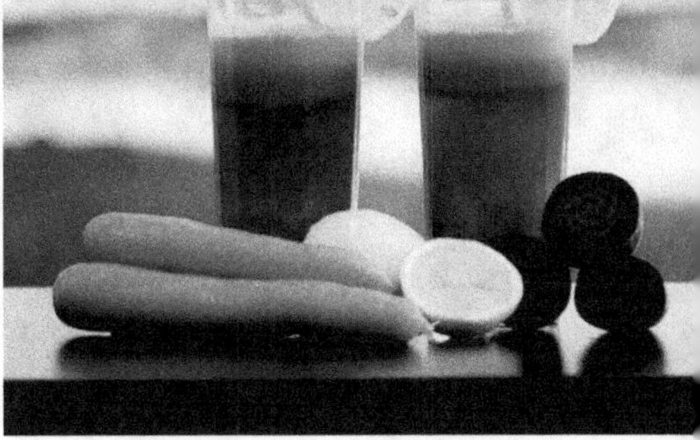

Carrot & Beetroot Eye Cleanser Smoothie

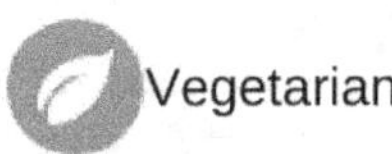 Vegetarian   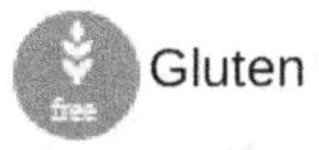 Gluten free   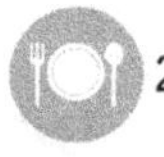 2 Servings   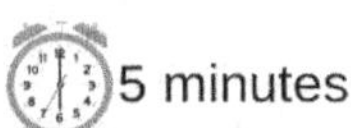 5 minutes

INGREDIENTS

- 2 large carrots,

- 1 small beetroot,

- 1 apple,

- 1 tablespoon hemp seeds,

- 1 cup of water.

Each sip promises hydration and a bounty of key minerals essential for maintaining eye health.

DIRECTIONS

1. Begin with the cool, crisp essence of 1/2 a cucumber, peeled and sliced,

2. Introduce the vibrant zing of 2 kiwis, peeled and diced,

3. Add 1/2 an avocado, peeled and pitted, its buttery flesh blending seamlessly into the mix.

4. Drizzle in a tablespoon of honey, nature's liquid gold, adding a touch of natural sweetness that complements the fresh flavors.

5. Finally, pour in a cup of coconut water, infusing the concoction with its subtle tropical notes and electrolytes,

6. Blend these ingredients to a velvety smoothness

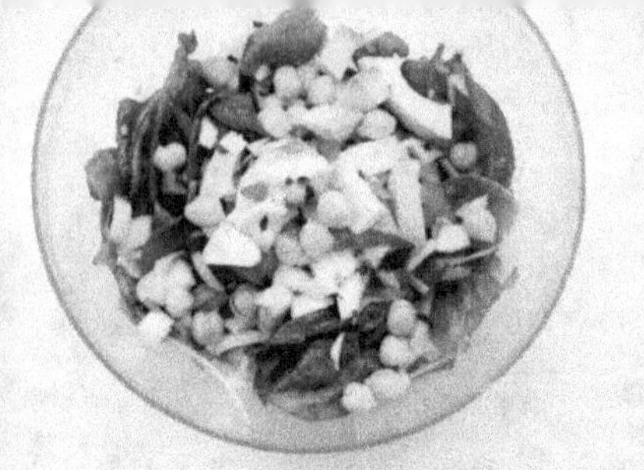
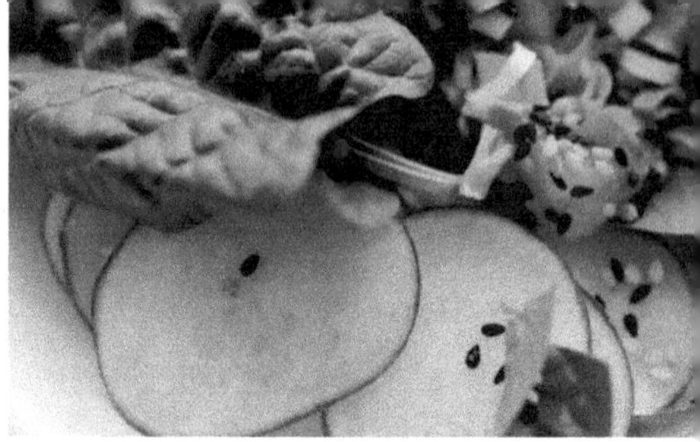

Tangy Spinach Salad with Mangos

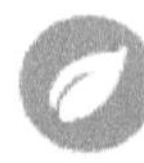 *vegans*    Gluten free   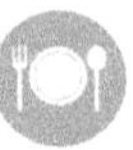 4 Servings    30 minutes

INGREDIENTS

- 2 perfectly diced ripe mangoes
- 4 cups freshly cleaned and dried spinach leaves
- 1/2 delicately sliced red onion
- 1/4 cup toasted cashews
- 1 spoonful of honey to balance the flavors;
- 2 tablespoons of extra virgin olive
- Juice of two freshly squeezed limes for a tangy twist.

This light salad is a taste explosion, with just the right amount of tart, sweet, and crunchy ingredients in each bite.

DIRECTIONS

1. First, prepare your mangoes by dicing them into uniform cubes.

2. Toss the roasted cashews, red onion slices, and fresh spinach leaves gently in a large mixing bowl to create a colorful salad base.

3. To make a rich dressing, combine the lime juice, olive oil, and honey in a different small bowl and whisk them thoroughly.

4. Over the spinach mixture, drizzle the zesty dressing and toss gently until all the leaves are uniformly covered and gleam with flavor.

5. Include the chopped mangoes in the salad and gently fold them in to evenly distribute the sweetness.

6. To ensure that the flavors blend nicely, let the salad sit in the fridge for approximately fifteen minutes.

7. Toss the salad one last time to reenergize the flavors just before serving. Enjoy the symphony of flavors in each bite by serving chilled.

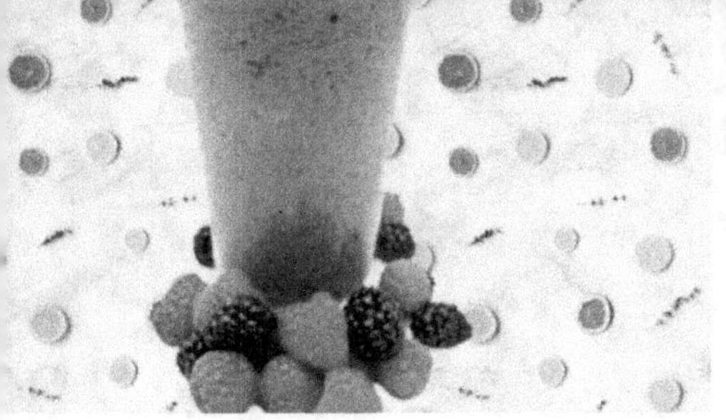
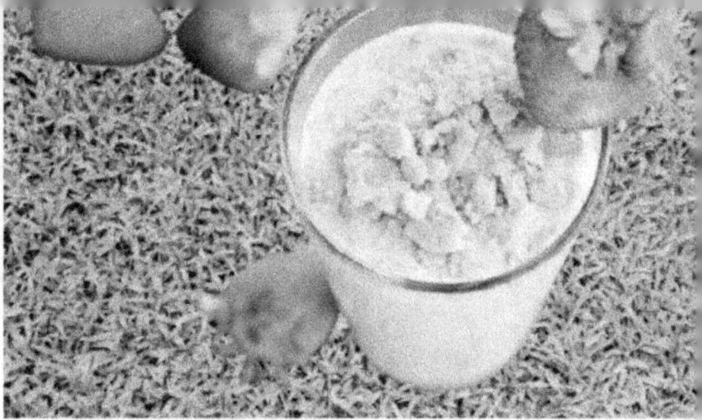

Berrylicious Blast Smoothie

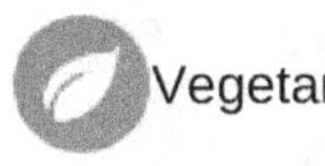 Vegetarian  Gluten free  1 Servings  5 minutes

INGREDIENTS

- 1 cup of frozen mixed berries

- 1 frozen and sliced banana

- 1 cup of unsweetened plant milk (oat, almond, etc.)

- 1 spoonful of chia seeds

- ½ cup baby spinach

Indulge in this high protein vegan blackberry smoothie. Perfect for a refreshing and nutritious snack

DIRECTIONS

1. In your trusty blender, combine all the ingredients.
2. Blend until the mixture achieves a creamy and smooth consistency.
3. Pour into your favorite glass and enjoy the berrylicious goodness!

Additional Tips

- *Adjust the amount of plant-based milk to your liking—more for a thinner smoothie, less for a thicker one.*

- *For an extra detoxifying boost, consider adding a small amount of kale or other leafy greens. Your taste buds and body will thank you!*

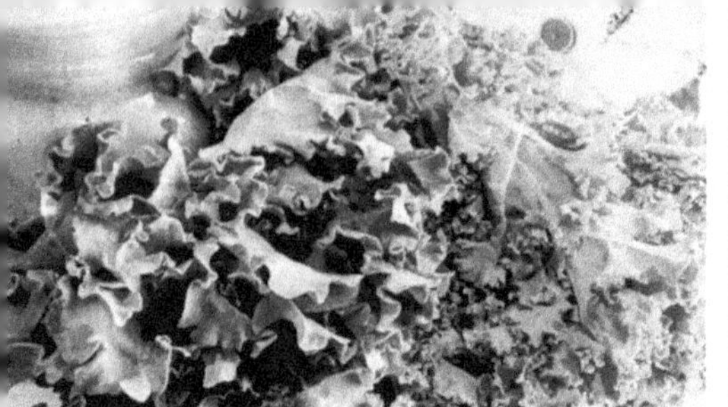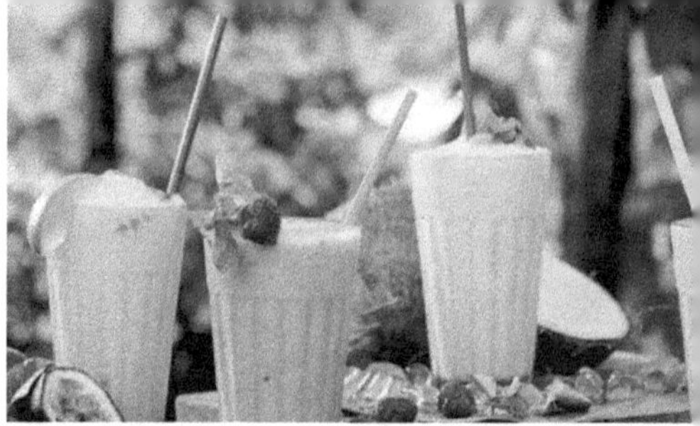

Tropical Green Dream Smoothie

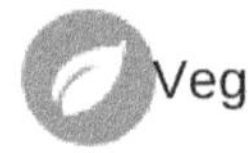Vegan 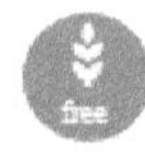Gluten free 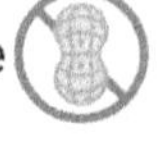Nut free 1 Servings 5 Mins

INGREDIENTS	DIRECTIONS

INGREDIENTS

- 1 cup of frozen or fresh mango chopped
- 1 cup of frozen or fresh pineapple chunks
- ½ cup of finely chopped kale
- 1 cup of plant-based milk without added sugar (coconut milk is suggested)
- 1 juiced lime

DIRECTIONS

1. Gather your ingredients—the sun-kissed mango, the golden pineapple, the verdant kale, and the luscious coconut milk.
2. Into the blender they go, like a harmonious tropical symphony. Blend until the mixture transforms into a creamy elixir, swirling with vibrant hues.
3. Pour into your favorite glass, and let the flavors dance across your palate.

- *Add an avocado or half an avocado for a creamier texture.*
- *To get the right consistency, you might need to add a little water or extra plant-based milk if the mango and pineapple are fresh.*

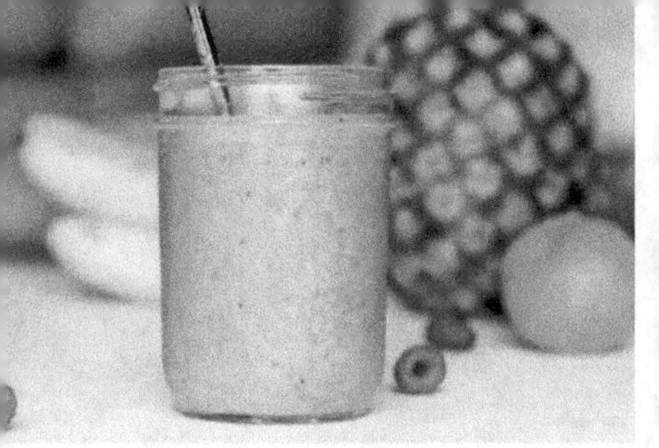
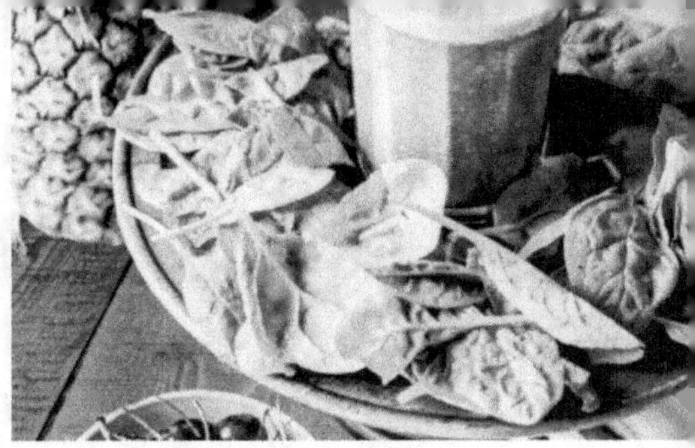

Spinach and Pineapple Eye Revitalizer Smoothie

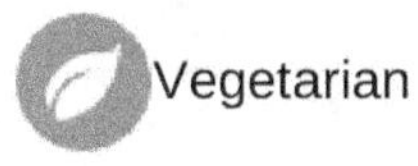 Vegetarian  Dairy free  2 Servings  5 minutes

INGREDIENTS

- 2 cups fresh spinach

- 1 cup pineapple pieces.

- 1 banana

- 1 tablespoon ground flaxseeds,

- 1 cup almond milk.

This smoothie is not just a feast for the eyes, but a revitalizing elixir, rich in vitamins and minerals, crafted to nourish your body and delight your palate.

DIRECTIONS

1.In a blender, combine a verdant oasis of fresh spinach leaves, two cups full, with a cup of succulent pineapple pieces.

2. Next, introduce the creamy, mellow tones of a ripe banana, Sprinkle in a tablespoon of ground flaxseeds.

3. Pour in a cup of almond milk, to unite the diverse chorus of ingredients.

4. Let the magic happen. Blend these treasures together until they reach a lusciously creamy consistency.

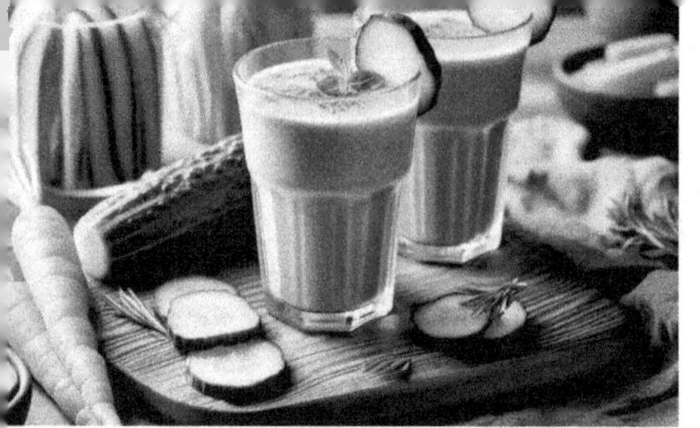
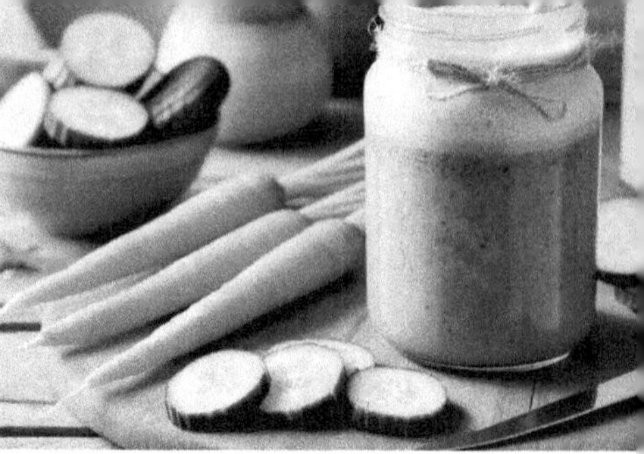

Eye-Bright Booster Smoothie

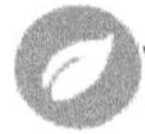 Vegan 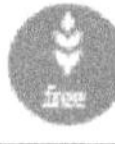 Gluten free 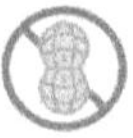 Nut free 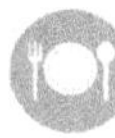 1 Servings  5 mins

INGREDIENTS

- 1 cup of chopped carrots, vibrant and full of beta-carotene

- 1 medium orange, divided and peeled

- ½ cup finely sliced cucumber, crisp and refreshing, like a cool breeze for your taste buds.

- 1 cup of plain yogurt, creamy and comforting, ready to embrace the other ingredients.

- ½ cup of cold green tea, a sip of tranquility that complements the medley.

DIRECTIONS

1. Assemble your ingredients—the orange, the carrot, the cucumber, and the yogurt.
2. Into the blender they go, like a harmonious orchestra tuning up. Blend until the mixture transforms into a velvety elixir, swirling with vibrant hues.
3. Pour into your favorite glass, and take a moment to appreciate the symphony of flavors.

Extra Tips

- *Add a pitted date or a sprinkle of honey for a sweeter smoothie.*

- *If preferred, you can use orange juice in place of the green tea.*

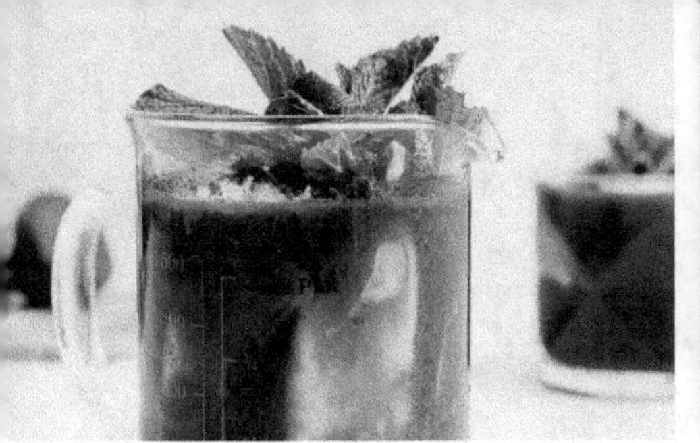
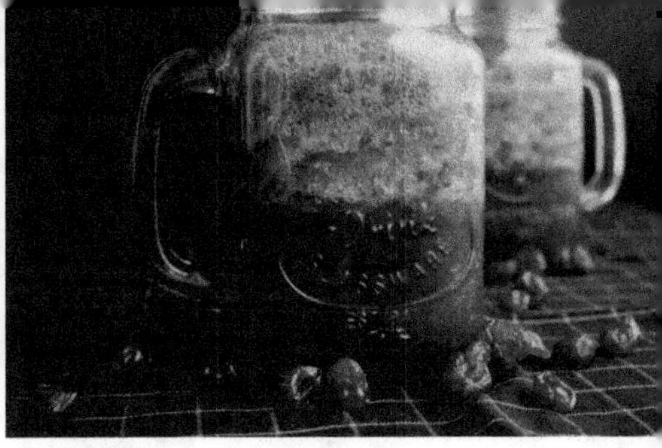

Beetroot Berry Blast Smoothie

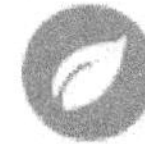 Vegan   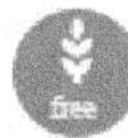 Gluten free   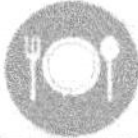 1 Servings    5 minutes

INGREDIENTS

- 1 medium-sized beetroot, cut and peeled,

- 1 cup of frozen mixed berries, a symphony of blueberries, raspberries, and strawberries,

- 1 cup of unsweetened plant-based milk, especially potent when it's beetroot milk,

- ½ a cup finely chopped beet greens (optional),

- 1 spoonful of flaxseed meal, these tiny seeds packed with omega-3 magic.

DIRECTIONS

1. Gather your ingredients—the beetroot's ruby allure, the berry medley's frozen charm, the milk's creamy promise, and the flaxseed's nutty secret.

2. Into the blender they go, like a botanical ballet. Blend until the mixture transforms into a velvety elixir, swirling with vibrant hues.

3. Pour into your favorite glass, and let the flavors pirouette across your palate.

- *When handling and cleaning beetroot, exercise caution since it can stain. Treat it like a precious gem.*

- *Beetroot greens taste strongly of earth, yet they are a fantastic source of vitamins and minerals. If you're feeling adventurous, toss them in. If not, skip the greens and savor the berrylicious bliss!*

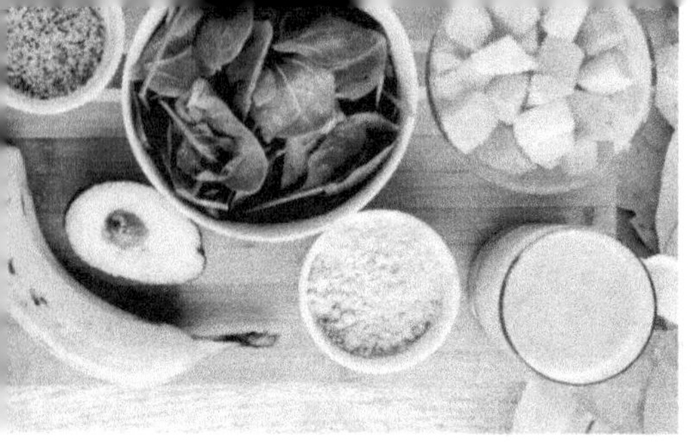

Green Power Smoothie

 Vegan  Gluten free 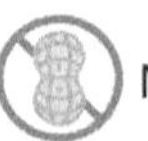 Nut free  1 Servings 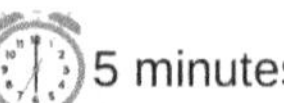 5 minutes

INGREDIENTS

- 1 cup of finely chopped kale,
- 1 cup of finely chopped spinach,
- 1 green apple, cored and chopped,
- 1 cucumber, peeled and chopped,
- 1 cup of unsweetened plant-based milk,
- Ripe banana (fresh or frozen).

For an extra boost, consider adding a sprig of mint or a squeeze of lemon.

DIRECTIONS

1. Gather your ingredients—the kale, the spinach, the apple, the cucumber, banana and the milk,
2. Into the blender they go, like a symphony tuning up. Blend until the mixture transforms into a velvety elixir, swirling with vibrant hues.
3. Pour into your favorite glass, and let the flavors dance across your palate.

- *You can substitute these to customize your recipes:*
- *Kale – If you're out of spinach, swap it with kale. Kale brings a robust earthiness and a boost of nutrients to your smoothie.*
- *Water – When plant-based milk isn't an option, water is your trusty companion. It hydrates without overpowering the other flavors.*

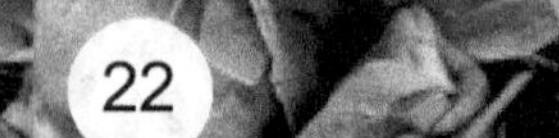

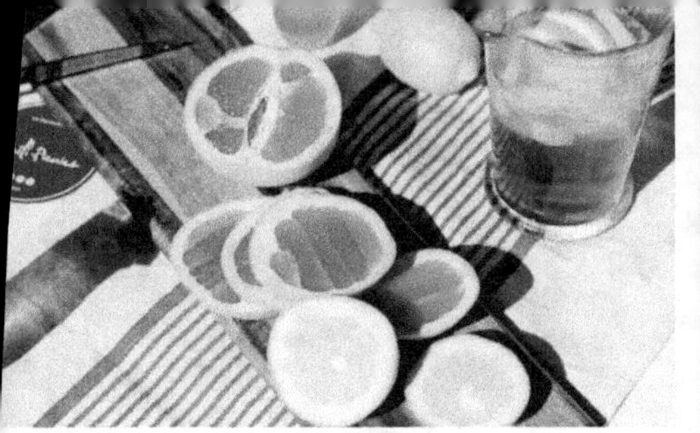
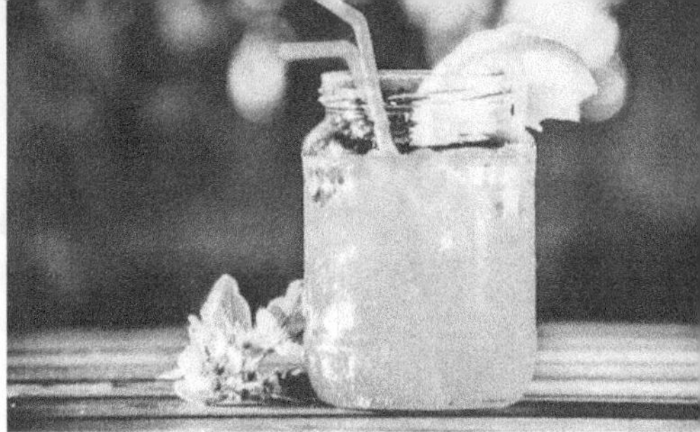

Citrus Sunshine Smoothie

 Vegan  Gluten free  1 Servings  5 minutes

INGREDIENTS

- 1 peeled and segmented grapefruit

- 1 peeled and segmented orange

- 1 lemon, cut into segments and peel (seed removed)

- ½ cup of pineapple, chopped

- 1 cup of plant-based milk, unsweetened.

DIRECTIONS

1. The grapefruit, the orange, the lemon, and the tropical touch of pineapple. Combine these with creamy milk for a symphony of flavor.

2. Whirl the ingredients together until a lusciously smooth blend is achieved.

3. Savor this delightful concoction as you pour it into a glass and enjoy the citrusy flavors.

Each sip carries the promise of vitamin C, nourishment, and a fresh start to your day.

- *Vitamin C, which is vital for general health, is abundant in citrus fruits. But you might want to cut back on the amount of lemon or grapefruit in this recipe if you have sensitive teeth.*

- *Water – When plant-based milk isn't an option, water is your trusty companion. It hydrates without overpowering the other flavors.*

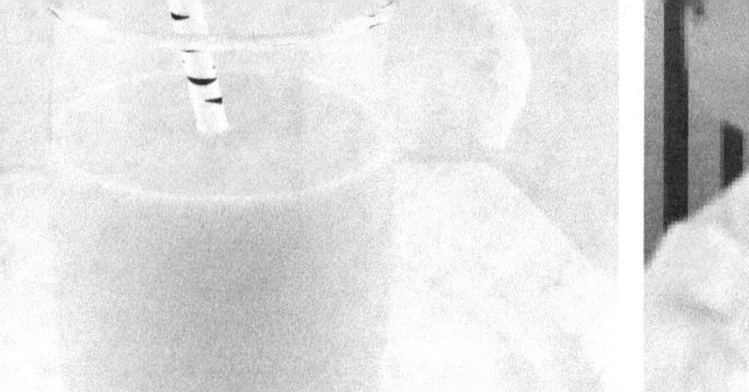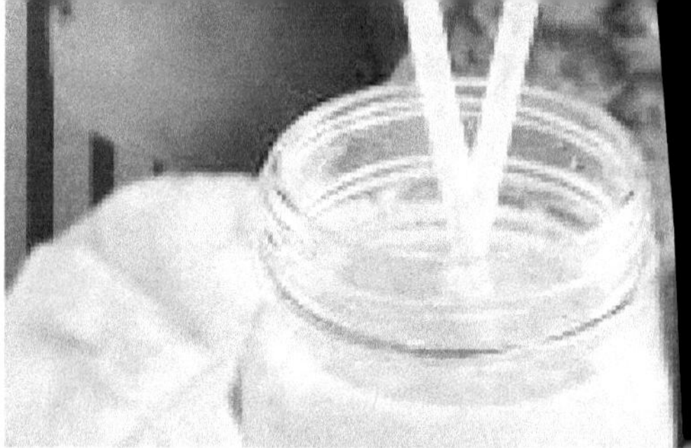

Ginger Zinger Smoothie

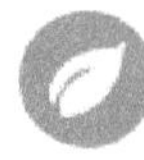 Vegan  Gluten free  1 Servings  5 minutes

INGREDIENTS

- 1 cup of frozen or fresh mango chopped,

- a 1-inch portion of peeled and chopped ginger,

- 1 cup of frozen or fresh pineapple chunks,

- ½ cup plant-based milk without sugar,

- 1 tablespoon of lemon juice.

DIRECTIONS

1. Gather your ingredients—the pineapple's zest, the ginger's kick, the banana's smoothness, the coconut milk's richness, and the turmeric's exotic flair.

2. Into the blender they go, like a tropical fiesta. Blend until the mixture transforms into a velvety elixir, swirling with vibrant hues.

3. Pour into your favorite glass, and let the flavors salsa across your palate.

Extra Tips

- *Due to its inherent anti-inflammatory properties, ginger may help lower optic nerve inflammation, which raises the risk of glaucoma.*

- *Because ginger has a powerful flavor, start with a tiny quantity and adjust the amount to your preference.*

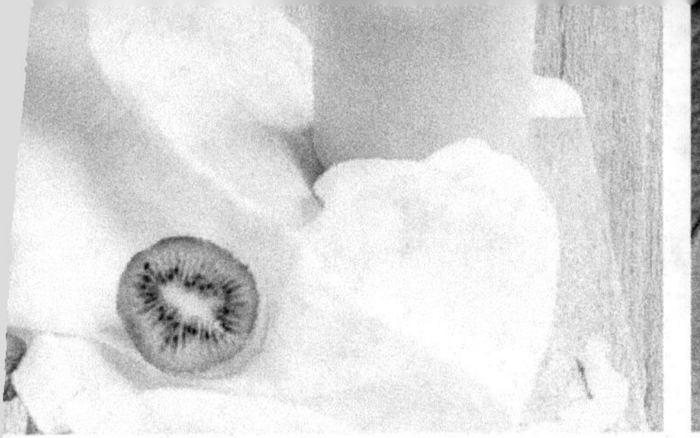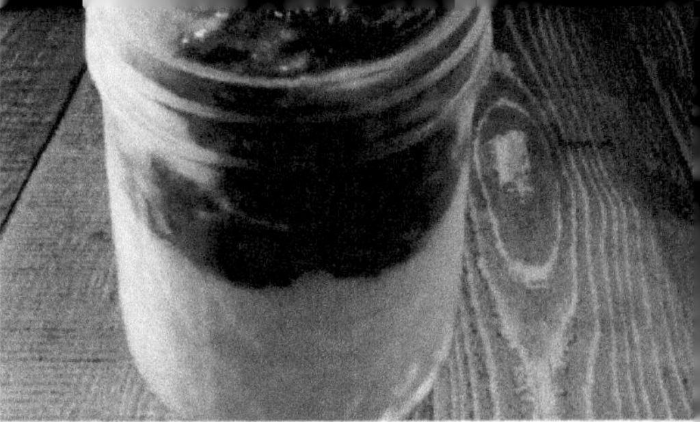

Tropical Turmeric Twist Smoothie

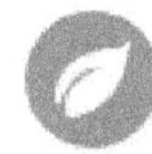 Vegan  Gluten free  1 Servings  5 minutes

INGREDIENTS

- 1 cup of frozen or fresh mango chopped
- 1 cup of frozen or fresh pineapple chunks
- ½ cup of finely chopped kale
- 1 cup of coconut water
- 1 tsp finely ground turmeric.

Extra Tips

- *Strong anti-inflammatory spices like turmeric may help lessen inflammation throughout the body, including the eyes.*
- *Turmeric has a strong flavor, so start with a small amount.*

DIRECTIONS

1. **Imagine this**: perfectly ripe mango chunks, bursting with juicy sweetness, dance with tangy pineapple in a creamy coconut water base. A hint of earthy, peppery magic from turmeric adds a surprising twist, leaving you wanting more. Finely chopped kale sneaks in some hidden greens, making this a guilt-free indulgence that nourishes your body.

2. Blend this tropical dream team until it's luxuriously smooth and creamy. Close your eyes, take a sip, and let the sunshine flood your senses. It's that good!

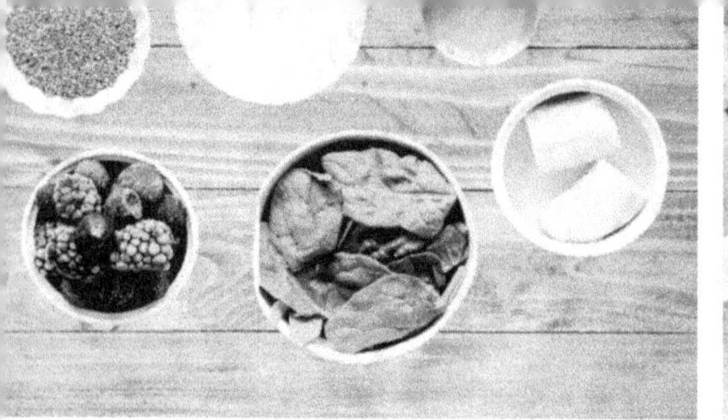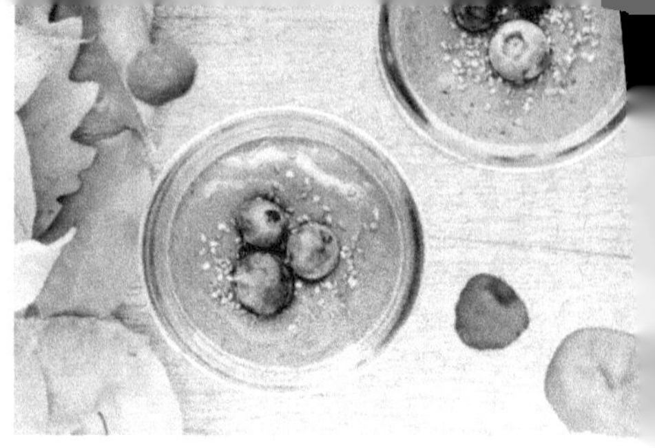

Superfood Seed Surprise Smoothie

 Vegan  Gluten free 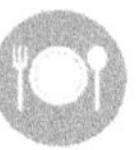 1 Servings  5 minutes

INGREDIENTS

- 1 cup of frozen mixed berries,

- 1 frozen and sliced banana,

- 1/2 a cup of finely chopped spinach,

- 1 cup of plain plant milk (almond milk is suggested),

- 1 tablespoon of chia seeds,

- 1 tablespoon of hemp seeds

DIRECTIONS

- Blend each ingredient until it becomes creamy and smooth. Give yourself a blast of tastefulness!

- *Omega-3 fatty acids are vital for general health and are found in both hemp and chia seeds. According to certain research, omega-3 fatty acids may aid in lowering inflammation and enhancing eye health, which is especially important for glaucoma patients.*

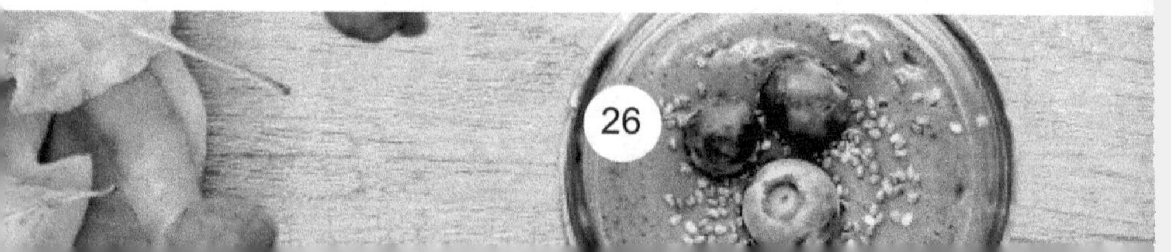

GREEN DETOX SMOOTHIES FOR GLAUCOMA

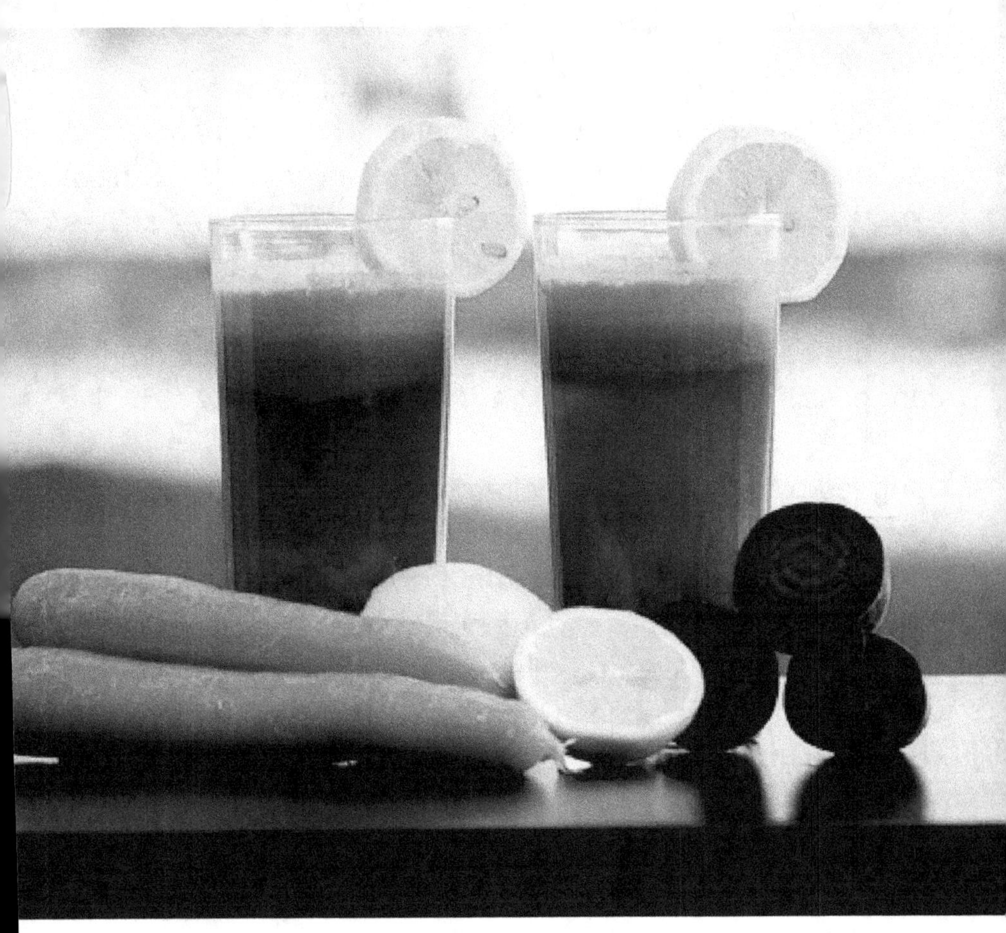

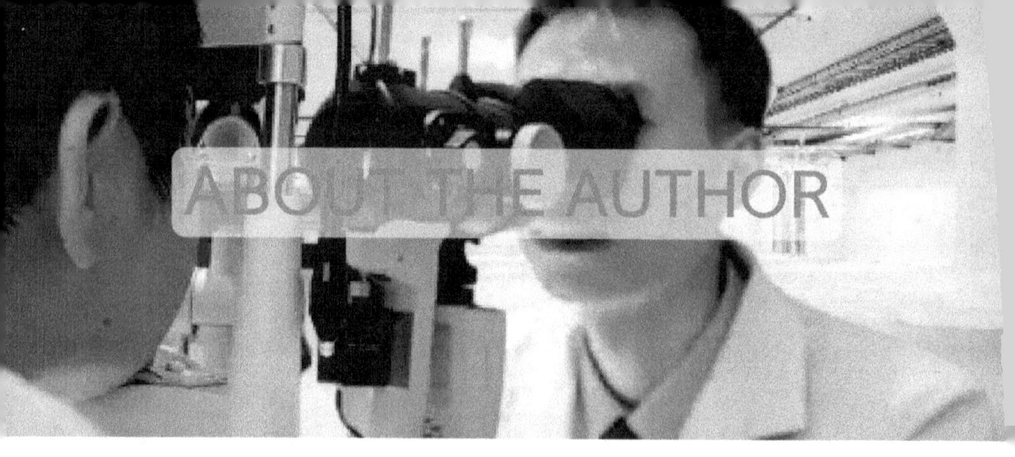

Dr. Ikukoyi Oluwaseun Akintan

Dr. Akintan isn't just an optometrist, he's a passionate advocate for your vision. With over eight years of clinical experience, his dedication to his patients' care shines through in every interaction. But Dr. Akintan goes beyond the ordinary. He's a constant learner, always pushing the boundaries of his field to bring you the most cutting-edge care possible.

Intrigued by the potential of alternative therapies, Dr. Akintan dives deep into the power of nutrition for eye health. This book is his exciting exploration of how food can complement traditional treatments, particularly for conditions like glaucoma. Dr. Akintan believes in empowering you, his patient, with knowledge. He doesn't just want to improve your sight, he wants to elevate your entire quality of life.

When you choose Dr. Akintan, you select a partner on your journey to optimal vision and a healthier you. Let him guide you with his expertise and unwavering commitment to your well-being.